Hughes Syn
The Antiphc
Syndrome

Graham Hughes • Shirish Sangle

Hughes Syndrome: The Antiphospholipid Syndrome

A Guide for Students

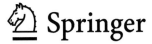 Springer

Authors

Graham Hughes, MD, FRCP
The London Lupus Centre
London Bridge Hospital
London
UK

Shirish Sangle, Associate Consultant
Louise Coote Lupus Unit
St Thomas' Hospital
London
UK

ISBN 978-0-85729-738-9   e-ISBN 978-0-85729-739-6
DOI 10.1007/978-0-85729-739-6
Springer London Dordrecht Heidelberg New York

British Library Cataloguing in Publication Data
A catalogue record for this book is available from the British Library

Library of Congress Control Number: 2011928405

Cover design: eStudioCalamar, Figueres/Berlin

Printed on acid-free paper

Springer is part of Springer Science+Business Media (www.springer.com)

Preface

In the quarter century since its description, the importance of the antiphospholipid syndrome (APS: Hughes Syndrome) has grown, the clinical ramifications of this major thrombotic syndrome now reaching into every branch of medicine. Yet despite its prominence as, for example, a major treatable cause of recurrent miscarriage, and as a preventable cause of stroke, it is still under-recognised.

A national "You Gov" survey commissioned by the charity Hughes Syndrome Foundation (www.hughes-syndrome.org) found that of over 2,000 adults questioned, only 4% had heard of the condition.

This short volume aims, from a very clinical perspective, to update practising physicians, medical students, health care workers and indeed all who come in contact with the condition, on the commonly recognised signs and symptoms of Hughes Syndrome.

Graham Hughes

Contents

List of Figures

Chapter 1
History

1.1 The Discovery

For me it started in Hammersmith and took off in Jamaica. In Hammersmith Hospital, our lupus team had a particular interest in brain involvement, and between 1971 and 1975, we published papers on antibodies which appeared to cross-react with the brain.

In 1975, I was posted "on loan" to the University of the West Indies to set up a rheumatology department in the hospital there. With me was a technician, Geoff Frampton, and a clinical research fellow, Wendell Wilson, a Guyanese doctor who stayed on after my year there to run the new unit.

We saw a lot of lupus and soon became intrigued with a group of young women who developed a form of spinal paralysis.[1] Interestingly, these patients had, in common, a positive lupus (ANA) test and a "false positive" test for syphilis, a finding also sometimes seen in lupus. We began to consider (possibly wrongly) the possibility that these "syphilis" antibodies (anticardiolipin) might cross-react with brain and cord phospholipids such as cephalin and sphingomyelin.

---

[1] A number of these cases had "Jamaican neuropathy", a disease now known to be caused by a retrovirus.

G. Hughes, S. Sangle, *Hughes Syndrome: The Antiphospholipid Syndrome*, DOI 10.1007/978-0-85729-739-6_1, © Springer-Verlag London Limited 2012

On my return to London we set up assays for anticardio-lipin antibodies and studied our rapidly growing lupus population at Hammersmith Hospital.

It quickly became clear that our patients with anticardio-lipin antibodies (aCL) had a number of important clinical characteristics.

Firstly, they had a propensity to clot – not just veins, but also, critically, arteries. The clinical picture, filled in on our clinic meetings and ward rounds, included recurrent miscarriage, strokes, memory loss, headaches, labile hypertension, livedo, Budd-Chiari, renal vein thrombosis, occasional thrombocytopenia, chorea, pulmonary hypertension and, rarely, catastrophic widespread thrombosis. We realised that the syndrome was not confined to lupus, but could – and frequently did – occur in isolation.

In 1982, I presented the syndrome to the Heberden Society of the British Society for Rheumatology, and in 1983, our first papers in the *BMJ* and *Lancet* were published. We initially called it the "anti-cardiolipin syndrome", but at the *1984* meeting of the British Society of Rheumatology, changed the name to "Primary Antiphospholipid Syndrome" (APS).

1.2 The Background

Some of the individual strands of what has become "the Antiphospholipid Syndrome (APS)" are to be found in the history of lupus. It is possible that one of the first case reports came from the great William Osler, who reported a male lupus physician with a stroke.

In 1906, Wasserman described the "reagin" reaction, one of the earliest autoantibody studies. In the 1960s and 1970s, the so-called lupus anticoagulant (LA) became widely studied, with cases of lupus patients reported with LA and abortion, as well as LA and thrombosis.

In the 1990s, it was found that the antibodies reacted not with simple phospholipids, but with a complex of altered phospholipids and so-called phospholipid-binding proteins such as Beta 2 glycoprotein and prothrombin.

Since 1983, the story has gained momentum, with a growing literature, with biennial international conferences and with inter-laboratory quality control studies.

Most of all, the syndrome is now recognised as a major cause of (young) strokes, of (mainly young) heart attacks, of migraine, of memory loss – and, of course, of thrombosis.

In the following chapters, I will briefly describe the effects of the syndrome on different organs.

Chapter 2
Hughes Syndrome:
The Clinical Features

The major clinical features are *thrombosis* – both in veins and in arteries, (the latter distinguishing Hughes Syndrome from most other prothrombotic disorders) – and *recurrent pregnancy loss*. The myriad of clinical features follow on from this tendency to "sticky blood!".

2.1 Pathogenesis

The disease is considered one of the *auto-immune diseases*, sometimes associated with other conditions such as lupus, but more often standing in isolation. Antiphospholipid antibodies (aPL) are very strongly linked to the clinical features of the disease. The mechanisms by which they cause the blood to clot are still unclear, though effects on platelets, on clotting factors and on endothelial cells have all been suggested.

Other mysteries remain: for example, what triggers a thrombosis in aPL positive individuals? And why, for example, if a "neurological" feature such as headaches or memory loss is due to blood clots and infarction, do the symptoms often resolve with anticoagulant treatment? Perhaps blood "sludging" is responsible in some cases of thrombosis. And do other influences play a role – genetics, smoking, diet, infection etc.? In many cases the answer is a clear "yes".

G. Hughes, S. Sangle, *Hughes Syndrome: The Antiphospholipid Syndrome*, DOI 10.1007/978-0-85729-739-6_2, © Springer-Verlag London Limited 2012

2.2 Vein Clots

A deep vein thrombosis (DVT), for example in the leg or the arm, is often the first manifestation. Studies from a number of major hospitals have suggested that positive aPL tests are seen in up to 20% of all DVTs coming into casualty departments.

Often the thromboses are major, and pulmonary emboli – sometimes fatal, are not uncommon. Recurrent pulmonary embolism may lead to some of the cases of *pulmonary hypertension* seen in a small number of patients with Hughes Syndrome.

Internal venous thrombosis can affect almost any organ, e.g., the eye, (retinal vein thrombosis), liver (e.g., Budd Chiari), kidney (nephrotic syndrome), adrenal (Addison's disease), and the brain (e.g., sagittal sinus thrombosis) (Fig. 2.1).

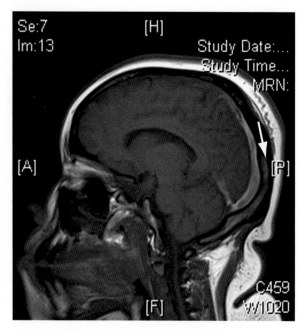

FIGURE 2.1 A CT angiograph of a brain showing sagittal sinus thrombosis in a patient with Hughes Syndrome

2.3 Artery Thrombosis

Cases can present dramatically, for example, with acute femoral artery occlusion leading to ischaemia and amputation. Vessels as big as the aorta can thrombose.

As with venous thrombosis, artery clots can lead to damage and failure in major organs such as the brain (stroke) and heart (myocardial infarction).

2.4 Pregnancy Loss

Failure of delivery of blood supply to the developing fetus can result in miscarriage. Hughes Syndrome is now recognised as the *commonest, treatable cause of recurrent pregnancy loss*. Tragically, some women suffer 8, 10, 12 and even more miscarriages before the diagnosis is made – a situation that could so easily have been prevented with simple aspirin or heparin.

On a positive note, research on the pregnancy aspects of Hughes Syndrome has contributed much to our knowledge of the disease – see Chap. 3.

2.5 The Brain

Of all the organs in the body, the brain seems particularly vulnerable in Hughes Syndrome. The clinical features of cerebral APS cover the whole of neurology, ranging from migraines, to stroke, to myelitis, to memory loss.

Indeed the syndrome is not only becoming a recognised important cause of stroke (e.g., 1 in 5 of all strokes in younger (under 45) individuals), but may come to be regarded as perhaps the major link between migraine and stroke.

2.6 Other Organs

Cardiac ischaemia is becoming recognised as an important feature in some cases of Hughes Syndrome (see Chap. 9).

As the story of the syndrome has unfolded, Hughes Syndrome has embraced all branches of medicine and surgery, including orthopaedics (ischaemic bone fracture), ENT (balance problems), dermatology (recurrent skin ulcers, livedo), psychiatry (memory loss) and transplant surgery (more complications in aPL-positive transplant patients).

Finally, somewhat bizarrely, low platelet counts can be seen, sometimes acute and severe, but more commonly in the 100,000 range (see Chap. 18).

Chapter 3
Hughes Syndrome: Pregnancy and Fertility

Recurrent pregnancy loss is one of the main complications of the Antiphospholipid Syndrome, with the losses ranging from early miscarriage to late fetal death.

Although there is some debate about the pathological process of the pregnancy loss, the predominant picture is one of extensive placental thrombosis and infarction (Fig. 3.1).

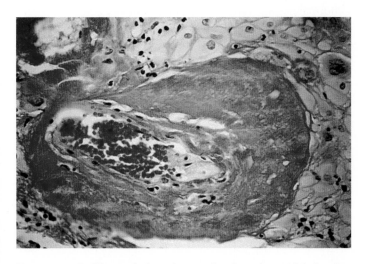

FIGURE 3.1 A Histopathology image showing placental infarction seen in Hughes Syndrome

G. Hughes, S. Sangle, *Hughes Syndrome: The Antiphospholipid Syndrome*, DOI 10.1007/978-0-85729-739-6_3, © Springer-Verlag London Limited 2012

Aside from placental ischaemia, other pathological mechanisms include aPL-mediated inhibition of trophoblast invasion, and placental inflammation.

3.1 Early Pregnancy Loss

Hughes Syndrome is now recognised as the commonest, treatable cause of recurrent miscarriage. Positive aPL tests are found in no less than 1 in 5 of women with recurrent pregnancy loss. Most of these losses occur before 3 months (at the present time, recurrent fetal loss is defined as three or more consecutive spontaneous abortions).

3.2 Late Pregnancy Loss

Tragically, later pregnancy loss can also occur in Hughes Syndrome. Other causes of pregnancy loss, such as chromosomal abnormalities, are much less common at this stage and, therefore, any woman with late pregnancy loss should be tested for aPL.

In the management of pregnancy in APS, Doppler measurement of fetal blood flow is a vital tool in assessing risk of ischaemia in the pregnancy, caesarean section usually being carried out when the Doppler starts deteriorating (Fig. 3.2a, b).

3.3 Other Pregnancy Complications

These include pre-eclampsia and placental insufficiency. For the mother, the risks of both venous and arterial thrombosis and intra-uterine growth retardation (and of thrombocytopenia) apply, as they also apply in the non-pregnant state.

3.4 Infertility

Some women suffering recurrent *very* early pregnancy loss have been diagnosed as infertile. This and other evidence, including unexplained implantation failure following IVF,

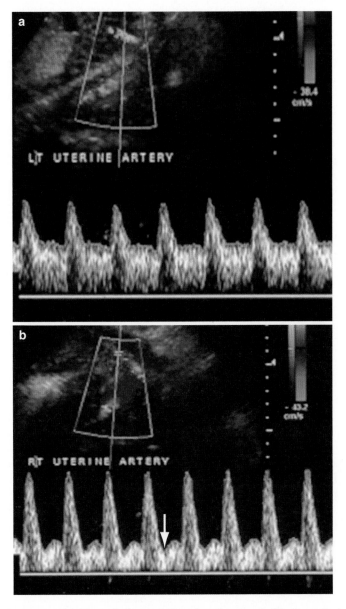

FIGURE 3.2 (a) Normal placental Doppler ultrasound. (b) A notched appearance seen (*arrow*) in placental Doppler ultrasound indicates placental ischaemia in Hughes Syndrome

has led to numerous studies of a possible role for aPL in the diagnosis and management of infertility.

The definition of infertility envisions a couple having frequent, unprotected intercourse, failing to conceive a child within a year.

The problem is common, affecting up to 20% of couples. Causes include hormonal, anatomic and possible immunologic factors.

Amongst the antibodies variously reported in infertility studies, aPL has been seen in 15–20%.

Whatever the mechanisms, these observations have led to studies of possible benefits of anticoagulation as a part of the IVF treatment regime. Early reports have been encouraging with those aPL-positive patients receiving aspirin or heparin having more than double the successful pregnancy rates – though other studies have failed to show this.

3.5 Treatment of the aPL-Positive Pregnancy

Anti-thrombosis treatment in aPL-positive pregnancy has proved to be one of the success stories of modern medicine, with pregnancy success rates improving from a previous under 20% to over 90% in most specialist centres.

Warfarin is contraindicated in the first trimester because of the risk of fetal malformation. The choice therefore is between low-dose aspirin and low-molecular-weight heparin.

Although physicians and obstetricians vary in their clinical practice, a general guide is taken from my colleague, Dr. Munther Khamashta, who has extensive experience in the management of pregnancy in lupus and APS.

Aspirin alone for an aPL-positive woman with no previous miscarriages, low-molecular-weight heparin plus or minus aspirin for those with previous thrombosis and one or more previous miscarriages (a disputed area – some would wait for two or more miscarriages before resorting to heparin).

Chapter 4
Venous Thrombosis

4.1 Venous Thrombosis and Hughes Syndrome

It has been estimated that in up to 20% of all cases of deep venous thrombosis (DVT) being admitted through casualty departments have the underling prothrombotic condition APS.

This makes it the commonest prothrombotic cause yet identified, commoner, for example than the association with Factor V Leiden. (It should also be remembered that APS, unlike factor V Leiden, can also lead to *arterial* thrombosis; see Chap. 10.)

4.2 Peripheral DVT

Leg and pelvic DVT remain the commonest presentations, sometimes clearly triggered by additional risk factors such as the oral contraceptive pill, or prolonged immobilisation, e.g., surgery, long-haul flights.

Axillary vein thrombosis is also seen – and should especially lead to testing for aPL (Fig. 4.1).

G. Hughes, S. Sangle, *Hughes Syndrome: The Antiphospholipid Syndrome*, DOI 10.1007/978-0-85729-739-6_4, © Springer-Verlag London Limited 2012

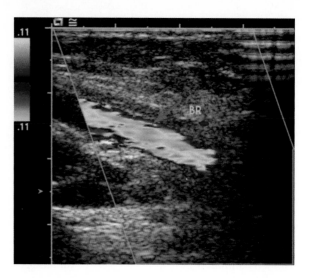

Figure 4.1 Color Doppler showing a clot in the axilliary vein (indicated by the arrow)

4.3 Leg Ulceration

Thrombosis in the leg can lead to leg ulceration, and Hughes Syndrome is now recognised as a cause of chronic leg ulceration – sometimes relieved with anticoagulation.

4.4 Pulmonary Embolism

Possibly because of the intensity of the clotting process in some cases of Hughes Syndrome, pulmonary embolism (PE) is not uncommon and is potentially a life-threatening complication of the syndrome – being reported in 2.1% of the 1,000 "Euro lupus" series of cases. Classically, PE presents with sudden chest pain, dyspnoea and collapse, though many varying symptoms can be found – including the well-known "urgent call for the bed pan".

One interesting paper studied the incidence and presentation of PE in passengers arriving by long-haul flights into

Charles de Gaulle airport in Paris. A common presentation was of the onset of symptoms *not* in the plane, but in the area between the plane and the customs hall – often with fainting preceding collapse. The authors attribute the timing to a moving of the clot (e.g.,a leg or pelvic thrombosis) after the traveller had stood and started walking.

4.5 Pulmonary Hypertension

One of the (fortunately uncommon) complications of Hughes Syndrome is pulmonary hypertension, a life-threatening condition in which the pressure in the pulmonary artery exceeds 25 mm of mercury. There are numerous causes of pulmonary hypertension (see Chap. 15), but "thromboembolic disease" is one recognised cause. Because the clotting and obstructive process in the lung can take years, it is difficult to be sure of the strength of the association between Hughes Syndrome and pulmonary hypertension. For example, in our series of cases with the combination, a small number of patients had been found to have a false-positive test for syphilis many years earlier – possibly due to aPL.

4.6 Trousseau's Syndrome

It has long been known that some malignancies, especially adenocarcinomas of the bowel, could lead to venous thrombosis. Not surprisingly perhaps, a few cases of Trousseau's syndrome have been described with positive aPL tests.

4.7 Organ Involvement

4.7.1 Kidney

Renal vein thrombosis is a recognised feature of Hughes Syndrome. It classically presents as acute or subacute loin pain, soon followed by proteinuria (often nephrotic), and ultimately, to renal impairment.

4.7.2 Eye

Central retinal vein thrombosis classically presents acutely with unilateral visual impairment or loss. It can be the presenting manifestation of the syndrome.

4.7.3 Liver

Intra-hepatic venous thrombosis is probably an under-diagnosed feature of Hughes Syndrome manifest by abnormal liver enzymes (for example in an aPL-positive lupus patient: abnormal liver function tests are rarely due to the lupus itself). More major venous thrombosis can affect the hepatic vein and the hepatic portal veins.

Budd-Chiari Syndrome (see Chap. 16) (hepatic vein occlusion – leading to ascites, jaundice, hepatomegaly and portal hypertension) was one of the features in the first descriptions of Hughes Syndrome in 1983.

4.7.4 Brain

Sagittal sinus thrombosis, presenting with headaches and visual disturbance, and manifest by raised intra-cranial pressure, has been described in a number of patients (see Fig. 2.1).

4.7.5 Adrenal

Adrenal vein thrombosis – because of the unusual adrenal blood supply pattern – can lead to adrenal infarction and Addison's disease (see Fig. 4.2).

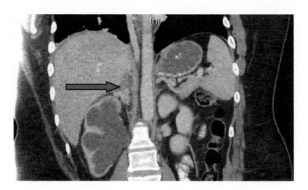

FIGURE 4.2 Magnetic Resonance Imaging scan showing adrenal infarction in Hughes Syndrome

Chapter 5
Migraine and Stroke

Did you suffer from severe headaches or migraines as a child or teenager?

"Yes, doctor.......severe, I missed a lot of school".

So often, on taking the past medical history in a patient with Hughes Syndrome, a story of teenage migraine comes out – often familial, sometimes disappearing only to return later, say, in their 30s or 40s.

5.1 How Frequent Is Migraine in Hughes Syndrome?

One of the problems which bedevil migraine studies – especially retrospective studies – is that of definition. There are numerous types of headaches and of migraines – not to mention abdominal migraine and balance problems. Despite this, it seems clear that the true strength of the association is strong. More worryingly, in patients with Hughes Syndrome, increasingly severe and frequent migraines can pre-date a TIA or stroke.

The aetiology of the headaches is also uncertain. The rapid response of many patients to anticoagulation with heparin or warfarin suggests that actual cerebral infarction is unlikely.

It seems possible that Hughes Syndrome might provide clues for those working in migraine research. It has been estimated that the annual cost of migraine in the USA is $17

G. Hughes, S. Sangle, *Hughes Syndrome: The Antiphospholipid*   19
Syndrome, DOI 10.1007/978-0-85729-739-6_5,
© Springer-Verlag London Limited 2012

billion. There is also a sizeable literature linking migraine with vascular events such as heart attack and stroke.

It may well be that aPL plays a major role in that link.

5.2 TIA and Stroke

Stroke and myelitis are probably the two most severe complications of APS. The whole spectrum of cerebral ischaemia can be seen in Hughes Syndrome, ranging from transient ischaemic attacks (TIA) (sometimes blurring clinically with hemiplegic migraine), through to multi-infarct dementia in untreated cases (Fig. 5.1).

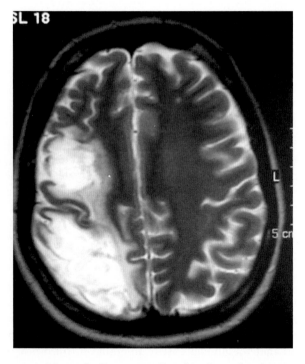

Figure 5.1 Magnetic Resonance Imaging Scan showing massive thrombosis in the right hemisphere of the brain in a patient with Hughes Syndrome

Symptoms range from sudden speech disturbance, through to balance problems, hemiplegic weakness, and in severe cases, worsening memory loss.

5.3 Stroke and Hughes Syndrome: How Common?

Soon after reporting the association in the early 1980s, we carried out a collaborative screening survey with colleagues in a large medical centre in Barcelona. We found aPL positivity in 7% of all strokes (including, of course, all major causes such as hypertension). Many epidemiological studies followed. Perhaps the most striking was a study from Rome which looked at *young* strokes – aged 45 and under. In this group, they found that APS was a possible aetiology in no less than 1 in 5 of all cases!

The cost – both economic and personal – of stroke is enormous. The possibility that a simple blood test – aPL – could screen out a significant (younger) subgroup in whom prevention would be possible is both exciting and tantalising.

5.4 Diagnosis

In clinical practise, brain MRI is the preferred investigation. In patients with multiple small infarcts, the lesions show as numerous small "dots" ("the sky at night") (Fig. 5.2).

However, there are two main caveats in interpretation.

Formerly, it was common practice to accept a few MRI "dots" as the normal process of ageing.

However, a seminal study from Holland, reviewing a decade-long collection of data, showed that such microlesions were *not* so benign and could progress to more widespread cerebrovascular disease.

The other caveat concerns the "normal" MRI. Many cases in whom unequivocal evidence of neurological injury is present have normal MRI. Clearly the current MRI has *some* limitations. The advent of PET, SPECT and other screening

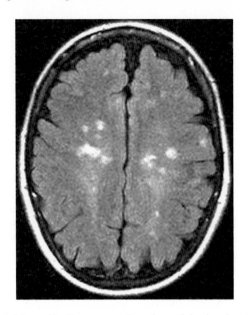

FIGURE 5.2 Magnetic Resonance Imaging of brain showing high density signals suggesting ischaemic lesions in a patient with Hughes Syndrome

advances are not yet here – at least not in the average hospital radiology department.

In summary, stroke is an important complication of Hughes Syndrome. The saving in both financial and human cost of a screening program for aPL in suspected T.I.A. or early stroke in a population for under 50 year olds must surely be significant.

Chapter 6
Movement Disorders and Seizures

6.1 Chorea (St. Vitus Dance)

The original description of the syndrome included a number of cases of chorea. We felt that this feature had a poor prognosis, as most of our cases went on to develop stroke.

The clinical picture of the chorea – with the writhing "Thai-dancing" movements of the hands – is classical. It is often misdiagnosed as being part of rheumatic fever (a condition which has been virtually absent from UK wards for 50 years).

However, it has one very important difference from rheumatic chorea – it often improves with anticoagulation.

Interestingly, chorea was the first neurological feature of Hughes Syndrome in which we observed an improvement on anticoagulation – suggesting perhaps more a "sludging" than a clotting of cerebral or basal ganglial blood flow.

6.2 Fits and Jerks

Neurologists now recognise a broad constellation of movement disorders in Hughes Syndrome. These range from sudden jerking movements of the arms, or of the head, through to a variety of continuous movement disorders (Fig. 6.1).

G. Hughes, S. Sangle, *Hughes Syndrome: The Antiphospholipid Syndrome*, DOI 10.1007/978-0-85729-739-6_6,
© Springer-Verlag London Limited 2012

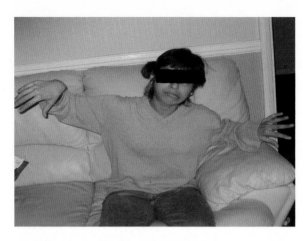

FIGURE 6.1 Extra pyramidal movement disorder in a patient with Hughes Syndrome

A small number of cases of Parkinson's disease have been recorded in association with aPL. Whether this will turn out to be an important association statistically remains to be seen.

6.3 "Mad Cow" Disease

Undoubtedly, the most dramatic case of movement disorder in my own experience was that of a farmer's wife from Durham, in the North of England.

She developed severe, widespread movement disorder, jerks, muscle spasms and varying spasticity. As this occurred at the height of the BSE, "mad cow disease" scare in the United Kingdom, she was fully investigated for this, with negative results. However, her neurologist checked her for aPL, which were found positive in high titre. She was treated with warfarin with total resolution of the neurological features.

Interestingly, she was one of a number of cases of Hughes Syndrome with cerebral features who required more vigorous anticoagulation. When the INR fell below 3.7, neurological features returned!

6.4 Epilepsy

Seizures have long been recognised as a feature of lupus. With the development of aPL testing, we found that it was mainly the aPL-positive lupus patients who suffered the seizures.

We now know that epilepsy – in all its forms, from Jacksonian, to petit mal, to temporal lobe epilepsy, are important features of Hughes Syndrome, so much so that EEG testing is now recognised as a vital tool in the investigation of APS (Fig. 6.2a, b).

How strong is the association? We don't yet know. However, in a recent careful study from Milan, the workers tested for aPL in a large group of idiopathic (no trauma etc.) teenage epilepsy sufferers. They came up with that same striking figure – 1 in 5!

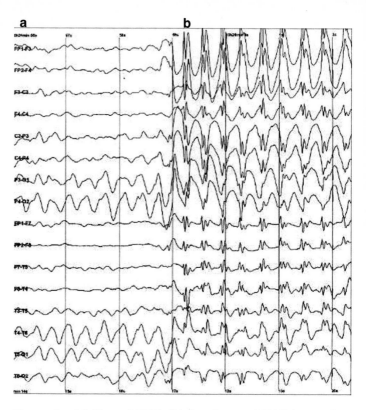

FIGURE 6.2 (a) Normal EEG. (b) An abnormal EEG in a patient with Hughes Syndrome showing high spiking EEG waves having seizure disorder in Hughes Syndrome

Chapter 7
Neuropsychiatric Aspects

7.1 Memory Loss

Many patients with Hughes Syndrome fear that they are developing Alzheimer's.

Memory problems are, like headaches, one of the commonest complaints in Hughes Syndrome.

The problems can take many day-to-day forms – slower with the crosswords or the Sudoku, for example.

Or difficulty in finding the right words: speaking obviously wrong words. Or the mother who could not remember which exit from the roundabout to take after dropping her child at school. Or the village darts champion who suddenly couldn't recognise the "20".

Clinicians who see patients with Hughes Syndrome have long recognised how big a feature this is in so many patients. Fortunately, neuro-psychiatric and psychometric studies are now emerging, confirming a wide range of abnormalities, ranging from decreased verbal memory to defects in psycho-motor speed and cognitive flexibility.

For a year or so, we were fortunate in having a senior research registrar from the department of psychiatry at St. Thomas's Hospital attached to our unit.

He undertook a number of psychometric assays (some taking hours!) on our volunteer patients. He never finally

G. Hughes, S. Sangle, *Hughes Syndrome: The Antiphospholipid Syndrome*, DOI 10.1007/978-0-85729-739-6_7,
© Springer-Verlag London Limited 2012

published his data but they certainly confirmed the findings in the literature.

With his permission, I mention on such study.

A young woman with Hughes Syndrome complained of memory problems – in particular, with word finding. She was often stuck for the right words – so much so that friends began to notice.

My colleague carried out a number of tests including IQ and word finding ability. The latter was poor........down at the 14th percentile.

As is our practice in some patients notably those failing to respond to aspirin, we tried a 4-week course of self-administered low-molecular-weight heparin. After the 4 weeks, a reassessment was made, including psychometry.

The results were striking (Fig. 7.1).

In four short weeks, her word-finding prowess had increased to normal – a finding verified by the patient herself. Our psychiatrists were intrigued – few psychiatric drugs ever give a positive result so emphatically.

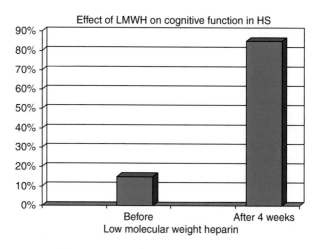

FIGURE 7.1 This graph shows improvement in cognitive function from 14% to over 80% in 4 weeks following LMWH therapy

This case reflects the observations made in many of Hughes Syndrome patients – the improvement in mental clarity ("the lifting of the fog") which often accompanies heparin or warfarin anticoagulation.

7.2 Other "Neuropsychiatric" Features

It seems entirely likely that, given the brain's myriad of responses to injury (including hypoxia), other neuropsychiatric features may dominate.

To date, the picture is unclear. Depression, for example, is a major feature of lupus: possibly not in Hughes Syndrome though. "We await further studies".

Certainly, anecdotal cases abound.

For example, in my clinic we have two families with multiple cases of Hughes Syndrome and obsessive compulsive disorder (OCD).

Co-incidence perhaps – or two separately inherited conditions – but in one of the patients there was striking improvement in the OCD when anticoagulation was started for a leg thrombosis.

We also have two families with strong histories of both Hughes Syndrome and autism. Again, coincidence or association?

Clearly there is room for far more in the way of psychometric and psychiatric studies to tease out some of the strands of the neurological syndrome – the temporal lobe epilepsy, the speech disturbance, and in some cases, the contribution of an associated condition such as lupus.

Chapter 8
Spinal Cord (Including Multiple Sclerosis) and Peripheral Nerves

8.1 Myelitis

Transverse myelitis is one of the most feared complications of Hughes Syndrome. Varying in severity from the localised, often fluctuating spinal cord features through to acute full blown paraplegia, the lesion is seen on MRI as a variable length ischaemic/inflammatory pattern (Fig. 8.1a, b).

As with epilepsy, myelitis has long been a recognised feature of lupus, and it is still uncertain in lupus patients as to how major a part aPL plays.

Common features are bilateral leg weakness, sensory level, bladder disturbance. There may be clonus and upgoing plantars.

The pathogenesis is still uncertain. Other antibodies are also being associated with myelitis, including Devic's disease – neuromyelitis optica.

Traditionally, at least in lupus, the emergency treatment for this potentially disastrous condition has been steroids and cyclophosphamide.

However, in view of the strong association with aPL, perhaps anticoagulation should be considered as well.

G. Hughes, S. Sangle, *Hughes Syndrome: The Antiphospholipid Syndrome*, DOI 10.1007/978-0-85729-739-6_8,
© Springer-Verlag London Limited 2012

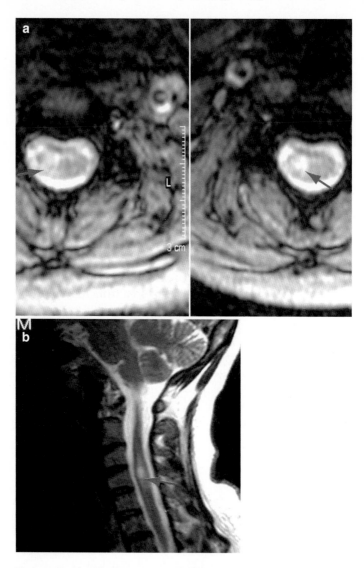

FIGURE 8.1 (**a**, **b**) Transverse myelitis in Hughes Syndrome; high density signals (white areas shown by *arrows*) indicate ischaemic lesions

One of my ablest research fellows, Dr. Aziz Gharavi, studied a mouse model of APS. Some mice developed paraplegia with spastic back legs. Histological examination of their spinal cords revealed.......thrombosis.

8.2 Multiple Sclerosis

In view of the wide spectrum of neurological manifestations of Hughes Syndrome, it is perhaps not surprising that some cases are originally considered to have multiple sclerosis (MS).

This differential diagnosis was such a recurring theme in our patients' histories that we carried out a standard questionnaire which included the question, "Did any of your doctors consider a diagnosis of MS in your case?"

The result was striking. Of those patients with positive aPL tests, 32% responded "yes", compared with 8% of aPL-negative patients.

The differential diagnosis can be difficult. In our studies, the clinical overlaps were considerable and the MRI (read "blind" by neuro-radiologists) were indistinguishable.

Clearly there is a need for further studies. How commonly does Hughes Syndrome masquerade as "MS"? How many Hughes Syndrome patients are currently being treated as "MS"? Is it 1%, or 5%, or more?

Important, as the treatments are very different.

8.3 Peripheral Neuropathy

As peripheral neuropathy is relatively uncommon in lupus, we were surprised at its frequency in Hughes Syndrome.

Again the clinical severity varies widely from mild sensory neuropathy to more severe generalised disease.

Interestingly, pressure neuropathy such as carpal tunnel (and perhaps some cases of "spinal stenosis", in aPL-positive individuals) are seen.

Perhaps there is a parallel with diabetes where partially ischaemic nerves are more vulnerable to pressure damage.

8.4 Autonomic Neuropathy

As might be expected, we have seen a series of APS patients with variable autonomic abnormalities. Perhaps we are missing milder cases.

8.5 Trigeminal Neuropathy

This appears not uncommonly in our Hughes Syndrome patients. Whether it reflects an ischaemic basis is uncertain. Cranial neuropathies were described in Sjögren's patients many decades ago; it is also possible that Sjögren's provides the common link.

Chapter 9
The Heart

If ever there was an "emerging market" for the Antiphospholipid Syndrome, it must surely be in cardiology.

After a slow start, where recognition of cardiac thrombosis in APS seemed to lag way behind cerebral thrombosis, the world of cardiology is now recognising its potential impact.

9.1 Heart Attack

A recent Lancet study (late 2009) found that women with positive aPL tests and starting the oral contraceptive pill had a 20-fold increased chance of myocardial infarction.

In another study, of 344 patients with acute coronary symptoms, approximately 40% were aPL-positive, and adverse effects occurred more frequently in the aPL-positive group.

The coronary thrombosis associated with aPL can attack at any age – one of my patients was a 21-year-old girl who died of acute MI while back-packing in Australia.[1]

The impact in cardiology may go much further. As well as an increased risk of coronary thrombosis, aPL-positive individuals have an increased tendency to re-thrombose after coronary surgery and stent procedures.

---

[1]In "Understanding" Hughes Syndrome. 50 clinical cases. Springer Verlag. ISBN: 978-1-84800-932-5.

G. Hughes, S. Sangle, *Hughes Syndrome: The Antiphospholipid Syndrome*, DOI 10.1007/978-0-85729-739-6_9, © Springer-Verlag London Limited 2012

One message is clear. Unexpected myocardial infarction in a young to middle aged woman should include the simple blood tests for aPL.

9.2 Syndrome X

One form of angina is referred to as "Syndrome X". The cardiac version of "Syndrome X" is one of angina with essentially normal coronaries on angiography. A number of patients with "Syndrome X" have been found to be aPL-positive – another potentially treatable condition, preventing more serious cardiac sequelae.

9.3 Pulmonary Hypertension

This severe condition, a result of thrombosis in some cases of Hughes Syndrome, is discussed in Chap. 15.

9.4 Valve Disease

One of the features of APS which distinguishes it from other clotting disorders is valve disease. This ranges in severity from mild valvular incompetence (mostly mitral) demonstrated in echocardiography, through to severe valve failure requiring surgery (Fig. 9.1).

At histology, the picture is one of a combination of adherent thrombus and mucinous degeneration of the valve.

Very occasionally the valve thrombus can reach significant size and cases of atrial myxoma have been described.

9.5 Patent Foramen Ovale

This topic is included more for discussion than from any hard evidence. However, it seems likely that thrombo-embolism in those patients with patent foramen ovale is bound to have more serious consequences including stroke.

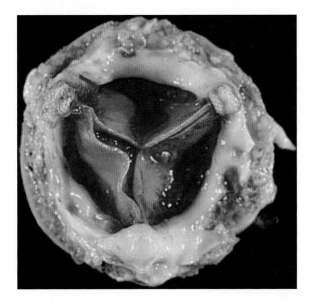

FIGURE 9.1 Heart valve abnormalities in Hughes Syndrome (Khamashta MA, *Hughes Syndrome: Antiphospholipid Syndrome*, 2nd ed., 2006, reproduced with permission from Springer Science+ Business Media B.V.)

9.6 Conclusion

Cardiac disease, especially cardiac ischaemia, is almost certainly about to become recognised as a major feature in some patients. While the pathology is based on thrombosis, it is possible that primary arterial disease may play a part. This topic is discussed next.

Chapter 10
The Arteries

One of the major features distinguishing Hughes Syndrome from other clotting disorders is the involvement of arteries.

The spectrum of arterial involvement ranges from acute obstruction, leading to infarction and gangrene, through the focal stenoses almost characteristic of Hughes Syndrome, to generalised "accelerated" atheroma, currently attracting the attention of researchers.

10.1 Peripheral Arterial Thrombosis

One of the bizarre features of the disease is the sudden – without warning – peripheral artery thrombosis – most commonly in the lower limb (Fig. 10.1).

One of my first patients with this presentation was the previously fit 19-year-old, rugby-playing son of the vice-chancellor of a UK university, who developed acute femoral artery thrombosis with peripheral ischaemia.

Arterial gangrene affecting the hands is unusual, though can be seen in patients with widespread "catastrophic" APS.

The unique picture of arterial thrombosis, seen in Hughes Syndrome, can even affect the aorta, and a number of cases of aortic arch syndrome mimicking Takayasu's arteritis have been recorded (Fig. 10.2).

G. Hughes, S. Sangle, *Hughes Syndrome: The Antiphospholipid Syndrome*, DOI 10.1007/978-0-85729-739-6_10,
© Springer-Verlag London Limited 2012

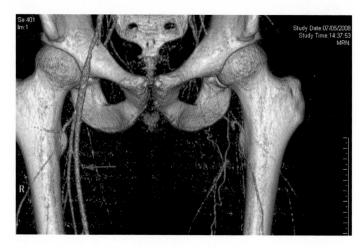

FIGURE 10.1   Right femoral artery occlusion in a patient with Hughes Syndrome. No femoral artery seen on the left side due to complete occlusion

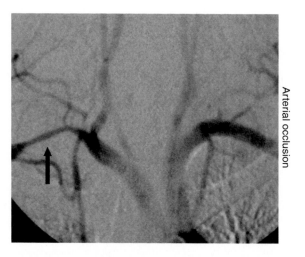

FIGURE 10.2   Right subclavian artery occlusion mimicking Takayasu's Disease in a patient with Hughes Syndrome

10.2 Internal Organs

Acute renal artery occlusion with renal ischaemia can be the presenting manifestation of APS.

Involvement of all major arteries has been described, including, of course, stroke, as well as retinal artery thrombosis, pituitary thrombosis, liver infarction, hip joint, gut (one of our patients presented with infarction of several feet of intestine) bone marrow and skin.

10.3 Focal Stenotic Lesions

These have now been described in many sites, including brain arteries, carotid, renal and celiac artery.

Renal artery stenosis, in particular, may be a prominent feature (Fig. 10.3).

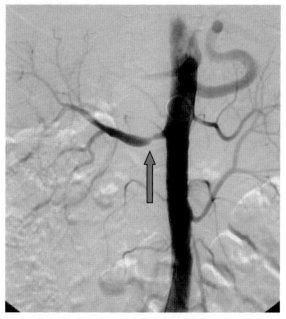

Right renal artery stenosis in Hughes Syndrome

FIGURE 10.3 Renal Angiogram showing right renal artery stenosis in Hughes Syndrome

FIGURE 10.4 Magnetic resonance
arteriogram showing celiac artery
stenosis in Hughes Syndrome

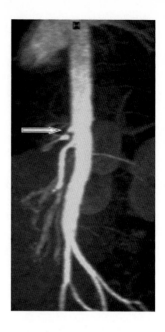

The stenotic lesions are completely different from those
seen in atherosclerotic disease and fibro-muscular hyperpla-
sia. They are localised, the remainder of the arterial tree
(including the aorta) being smooth and usually free from the
irregularities seen in atheroma.

Renal artery stenosis can lead to hypertension – to be discussed in the next chapter.

Whilst screening angiographically for renal artery stenosis,
we came upon another lesion – celiac artery stenosis (Fig. 10.4).
A number of these patients (though not all) suffered from the
classic features of mesenteric angina, with abdominal pain
following at an interval after a large meal.

The aetiology of these focal lesions remains uncertain, though localised thrombosis does appear to be the most likely cause. It is possible (though unproven) that such local lesions could lead to arterial wall weakness: Interestingly, a small number of cases of arterial aneurysm formation have been reported in association with APS.

10.4 Accelerated Atheroma

A topic of active research is the possible link between antiphospholipid antibodies and accelerated arterial disease.

It is well known, for instance, in lupus patients, that early onset arterial disease can be a major problem – so much so that lupus is sometimes referred to as the "new diabetes".

The causes of this feature remain uncertain – steroids, kidney disease and inflammation have all been looked at but none alone totally explains the link.

One line of research follows the observation that certain aPL can cross-react with oxidised low-density lipoproteins – a key player in atheroma formation.

Studies are in progress to assess whether aPL-positive lupus patients are more at risk from accelerated arterial disease.

An obvious question concerns the prevalence of this feature in APS patients (who have never taken steroids, who have no renal disease and who have no clinical evidence of chronic inflammation).

And, interestingly, initial studies do suggest early arterial disease in some of these patients – studies using indirect methods to look at arterial function, it must be said.

Chapter 11
The Kidneys

Perhaps because of the overlap of some cases of APS with lupus, recognition of the importance and extent of renal involvement in primary APS was initially slow. However, it is now known that a variety of renal pathologies can be seen.

11.1 Renal Artery Thrombosis

There are many reports of acute renal artery occlusion in APS – both unilateral and bilateral. Clinically the features include renal angle pain, haematuria, labile hypertension and, in some cases, acute renal failure.

Clearly an acute medical emergency, frequent options range from anticoagulation, through angioplasty to nephrectomy – the latter sometimes required for blood pressure control.

11.2 Renal Vein Thrombosis

Recognised in APS as well as aPL-positive lupus patients, renal vein thrombosis can be unilateral or bilateral. One of our cases presented post-partum with bilateral renal vein thrombosis and severe nephrotic syndrome.

G. Hughes, S. Sangle, *Hughes Syndrome: The Antiphospholipid Syndrome*, DOI 10.1007/978-0-85729-739-6_11,
© Springer-Verlag London Limited 2012

11.3 Renal Artery Stenosis

The original description of the syndrome included the observation, "these patients blood pressure often fluctuates, apparently correlating with the severity of the livedo, suggesting a possible reno-vascular aetiology. However, this group of patients rarely has primary renal disease".

We now know that renal artery stenosis underlies some of these cases (Fig. 11.1).

Studies of renal artery stenosis in APS found that, as might be expected, hypertension was a common accompaniment. This observation led to two others: firstly, that in APS, 80% of hypertensive patients were found to have livedo. And secondly, that in some APS patients, with renal artery stenosis, careful anticoagulation improves blood pressure control – another example of anticoagulation benefit in APS, even in the absence of overt thrombosis.

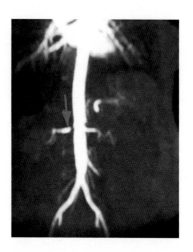

FIGURE 11.1 Magnetic resonance arteriography showing renal artery stenosis in Hughes syndrome

11.4 Thrombotic Microangiopathy

Glomerular thrombosis has long been recognised as a histological feature in some lupus kidney biopsy specimens. Indeed, careful studies have suggested that glomerular thrombi featured in up to 50% of lupus nephritis biopsies. It became clear that the association was with the presence of aPL, and in 1992, Amigo and her colleagues in Mexico reported the same pathology in primary APS.

Although thrombotic microangiopathy can be a result of a number of conditions, it is an important component of APS. In lupus, the search for aPL-related microthrombic lesions is now considered one of the main indications for renal biopsy.

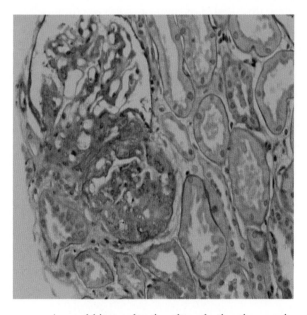

FIGURE 11.2 A renal biopsy showing thrombotic micro-angiopathy in a patient with Hughes syndrome. This young patient presented with hypertension, hematuria and impaired renal function

11.5 Renal Transplantation

The presence of aPL has long been recognised as a predictor of access thrombosis in dialysis treatment of end stage renal disease. Much more serious is the probable increased risk of failure of renal transplantation of aPL-positive individuals. Many published reports cite the higher rejection rate in aPL-positive individuals – not only in renal transplants – the problems largely being peri- and post-operative thrombosis.

However, for some patients, the prothrombotic risk continues for life and thrombosis in the transplanted organ can occur years after the surgical procedure.

Recognition of the thrombotic risk in APS and its appropriate management with anticoagulation has had a major impact in this branch of surgery, as it has in others.

To quote two transplant surgeons:

> *In the United States in 2003, the average cost of a kidney transplant was estimated to be $117,317. The expense of losing a transplanted heart or liver to aPL-associated thrombosis not only includes healthcare dollars but often includes the loss of a patient's life.*
>
> *The encouraging news is that once aPL are identified pre-transplant, prophylactic anticoagulation appears capable of averting aPL associated allograft event.* (Wagenknecht & McIntyre. Chapter in Hughes Syndrome. Ed. Khamashta MA. Springer).

Chapter 12
Skin

The commonest skin manifestations of APS are livedo reticularis and thrombotic skin ulcers.

12.1 Livedo Reticularis

This is one of the most important physical signs in APS and is felt by many physicians to be an additional risk factor for the risk of APS clinical events, over and above the presence of aPL (Fig. 12.1).

It has a characteristic blotchy appearance, described by one patient as "corned beef skin" and is most commonly seen on the knees, thighs, buttocks and the wrists. The livedo is a result of diminished blood flow from the deeper skin arterioles to the more superficial venules and capillaries. It is seen in a variety of conditions which affect inflow or outflow to skin vessels (including hyperviscosity syndromes). Dermatologists recognise two main forms, the pathologically significant form having an irregular, incomplete pattern (livedo racemosa). Histologically, the picture is one of obliterating vascular lesions, with no evidence of inflammatory vasculitis.

G. Hughes, S. Sangle, *Hughes Syndrome: The Antiphospholipid Syndrome*, DOI 10.1007/978-0-85729-739-6_12,
© Springer-Verlag London Limited 2012

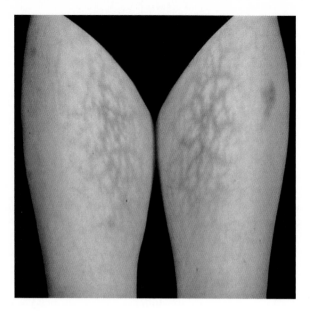

FIGURE 12.1 Livedo reticularis in Hughes Syndrome

The clinical severity can vary but it is interesting to note the improvement in livedo seen in many patients with Hughes Syndrome with effective anticoagulation.

12.2 Skin Ulcers

Skin ulcers are an important feature of APS with reports of up to 30% of APS patients developing ulcers – most commonly leg ulcers. They are presumed secondary to venous thrombosis, though in many cases there is no clear antecedent history of, for example, DVT.

They vary in size from ½ cm in diameter, through to large, necrotic leg ulcers several centimetres across. Clinical experience has shown that healing in many cases, though not all, is improved with anticoagulation treatment (Fig. 12.2).

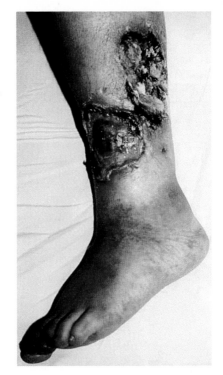

FIGURE 12.2 Cutaneous ulcer in Hughes Syndrome (Khamashta MA, *Hughes Syndrome: Antiphospholipid Syndrome*, 2nd ed., 2006, reproduced with permission from Springer

12.3 Digital Gangrene

This, a well-known complication of Hughes Syndrome, can follow either isolated arterial thrombosis or be a part of the more widespread thrombotic process seen in the catastrophic APS (Fig. 12.3).

12.4 Splinters

Subungual nail-fold infarcts are a prominent feature in some cases. They can be multiple (as in infectious endocarditis) and, strikingly, can be a recurrent feature pre-menstrually in some APS patients (Fig. 12.4).

FIGURE 12.3 Digital
Gangrene in Hughes
Syndrome,
(Khamashta MA,
Hughes Syndrome:
Antiphospholipid
Syndrome, 2nd ed.,
2006, reproduced
with permission
from Springer
(Khamashta MA,
Hughes Syndrome:
Antiphospholipid
Syndrome, 2nd ed.,
2006, reproduced
with permission
from Springer)

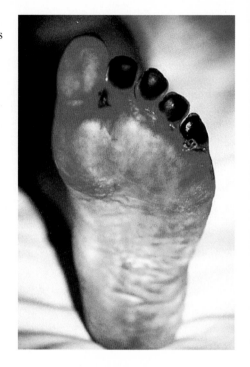

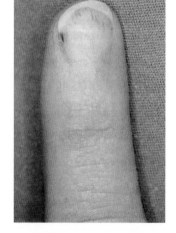

FIGURE 12.4 Splinter hemorrhage
in a fingernail in Hughes
syndrome

Chapter 13
The Eye

The eye is frequently affected in Hughes Syndrome. The commonest manifestations relate to ischaemic damage in the posterior segment, with retinal and choroidal lesions resulting from either arterial or venous thrombosis, or both.

The commonest symptom is of transient visual disturbance (transient blurred vision or amaurosis fugax) with diplopia and transient field loss a frequent complaint.

Clinical findings include venous engorgement, occluded central vein or artery and secondary haemorrhage. The ocular symptoms may also result from cerebral infarction in the occipital cortex, patients being left with, for example, permanent bitemporal hemianopia.

13.1 Optic Neuritis

A number of cases of optic neuritis have been described in patients with Hughes Syndrome, as have been cases of Devic's disease (neuromyelitis optica). This highlights the difficulties in differential diagnosis of Hughes Syndrome from multiple sclerosis (Fig. 13.1).

G. Hughes, S. Sangle, *Hughes Syndrome: The Antiphospholipid Syndrome*, DOI 10.1007/978-0-85729-739-6_13,
© Springer-Verlag London Limited 2012

FIGURE 13.1 A fluorescent angiography showing retinal hemorrhage and optic disc atrophy in a patient with both Hughes Syndrome and Devic's syndrome

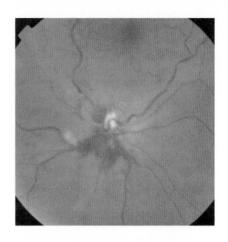

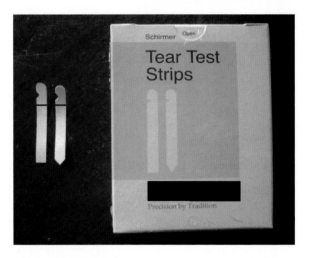

FIGURE 13.2 Patients with Sjögren's syndrome often have Sicca syndrome (dry eyes, mouth and vagina). This can be easily tested in eyes by Schirmer's test (see chap. 23)

13.2 Sjögren's Syndrome

As in many other autoimmune diseases such as Hashimoto's thyroiditis, there may be associated Sjögren's syndrome, with a dry Schirmer's test (impaired tear secretion) and a tendency to conjunctival irritability and infection (Fig. 13.2).

Chapter 14
Ear, Nose and Throat

One of the commonest (and possibly still under-recognised) symptoms of Hughes Syndrome involves balance and hearing problems.

In a number of patients, for example, the initial presentation of APS is of acute vertigo, often labelled as Meniere's disease.

Other balance problems are frequent, some associated with migraine.

Tinnitus is seen in a few patients.

14.1 Hearing Loss

Sensory neural hearing loss is a condition characterised by progressive hearing loss in previously healthy people. For the past 30 years, it has been labelled as possibly "auto-immune," a label based partly on experimental and histological studies as well as an association with various auto-immune disorders. There is a logical reason why APS might be implicated in some of these cases.

The cochlear vessels supply an end-organ and like the cerebral vessels, hip vessels and others, ischaemia here could result in loss of function.

G. Hughes, S. Sangle, *Hughes Syndrome: The Antiphospholipid Syndrome*, DOI 10.1007/978-0-85729-739-6_14,
© Springer-Verlag London Limited 2012

A number of studies of sensory-neural hearing loss have suggested an association with aPL, raising the speculation that this disease is microthrombotic (rather than inflammatory).

Chapter 15
Lungs

Pulmonary embolism, following a peripheral venous thrombosis, and in situ pulmonary thrombosis are well-recognised features of Hughes Syndrome (Fig. 15.1).

A second important complication of Hughes Syndrome is pulmonary hypertension (PHT). Although recognised in the original 1983 descriptions, the extent of the association is not yet known.

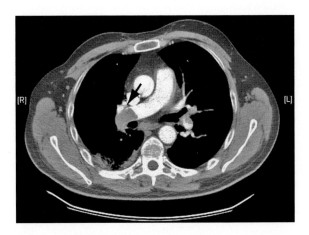

FIGURE 15.1 A CT pulmonary angiogram showing thrombosis in the right pulmonary artery in Hughes syndrome

G. Hughes, S. Sangle, *Hughes Syndrome: The Antiphospholipid Syndrome*, DOI 10.1007/978-0-85729-739-6_15, © Springer-Verlag London Limited 2012

15.1 Pulmonary Hypertension

PHT is defined as a mean pulmonary artery pressure greater than 25 mmHg. Although there are a number of recognised causes of PHT, (Fig. 15.2a, b) including genetic factors, chronic hypoxia, left ventricular failure and repeated pulmonary embolism, in the majority of cases of PHT, the cause is unknown.

Whether the process is predominantly of recurrent pulmonary embolism or of in situ pulmonary thrombosis is also unknown. The assessment of patients thought to have PHT has become the job of specialised cardiopulmonary centres.

Medical treatment includes anticoagulation, oxygen support, prostacyclin analogues and newer drugs including Bosentan (endothelial B receptor inhibitor).

Surgical treatment in severe cases can include thrombo-endarterectomy, septectomy and, in some cases, heart–lung transplantation.

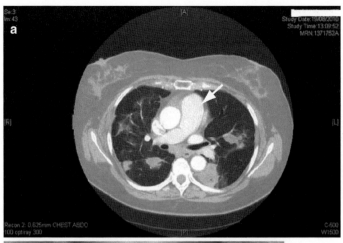

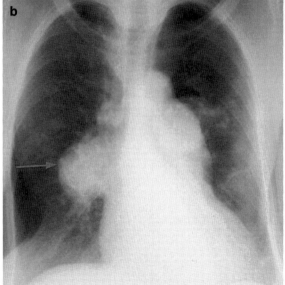

FIGURE 15.2 (**a**) and (**b**) A CT scan and chest X-ray showing dilated pulmonary vessels in a case of pulmonary hypertension in Hughes syndrome

Chapter 16
Liver and Gut

16.1 Liver

Hepatic artery thrombosis and liver infarction can occur in APS, as can hepatic venous thrombosis. Budd–Chiari syndrome (thrombosis of the hepatic vein) is a well-known sequel of APS, leading to hepato-splenomegaly (Fig. 16.1). One study

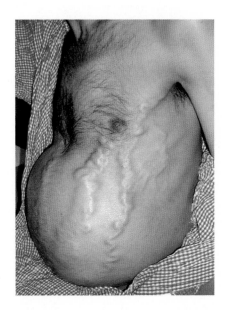

FIGURE 16.1 Hepatic Vein Thrombosis (Budd-Chiari syndrome) and collateral circulation in Hughes syndrome. Picture used courtesy of www.doctor-shangout.com

G. Hughes, S. Sangle, *Hughes Syndrome: The Antiphospholipid Syndrome*, DOI 10.1007/978-0-85729-739-6_16, © Springer-Verlag London Limited 2012

has suggested that Hughes Syndrome may be the second commonest cause of Budd–Chiari (second only to lymphoma).

Abnormal liver function tests are common in APS, and chronic liver ischaemia can lead to liver cirrhosis – a complication of APS whose frequency remains unknown.

16.2 Gut

A number of cases of bowel infarction have been reported, often requiring major surgery. Following the observation that renal artery stenosis is a feature of Hughes Syndrome, Sangle and colleagues in St. Thomas Hospital reported a substantial series of patients with celiac and mesenteric artery stenoses (Fig. 16.2).

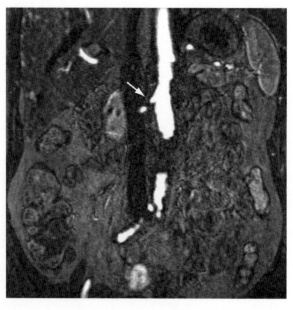

FIGURE 16.2 Magnetic resonance arteriogram showing superior mesenteric artery stenosis in Hughes syndrome

The clinical features in many cases were those of mesenteric angina – abdominal pain an hour or so after a large meal. (Not all cases were symptomatic, presumably due to the good vascular network of collaterals supplying the gut.)

As with the case of renal artery stenosis, a number of patients with celiac artery stenosis improved with thorough anticoagulation.

Chapter 17
Bones and Joints

17.1 Avascular Necrosis

A number of cases of "idiopathic" bone necrosis have been reported in aPL-positive individuals with no other risk factors and who have never received steroids. These include avascular lesions in the hip and shoulder, for example (Fig. 17.1).

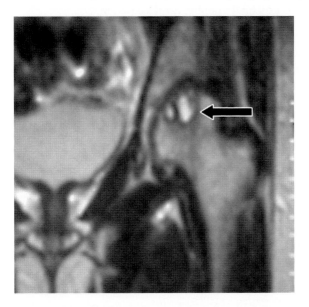

FIGURE 17.1 Avascular necrosis of hip in Hughes Syndrome

G. Hughes, S. Sangle, *Hughes Syndrome: The Antiphospholipid Syndrome*, DOI 10.1007/978-0-85729-739-6_17, © Springer-Verlag London Limited 2012

A large, multinational study of lupus patients with avascular necrosis (AVN) showed twice the incidence in aPL-positive individuals despite comparable steroid histories.

Despite these observations, the jury is still out on the overall contribution of APS to bone necrosis, some studies so far failing to find a significant link. Yet logically, the link makes sense. The hip joint, for example, is an end-organ, ischaemia or obstruction of the vascular supply to the head of femur having major consequences. This author believes that the link with AVN will prove a strong one.

An interesting clinical observation has come from the management of APS patients with hip pain. A small number have noticed pain relief in the hip when anticoagulation was started. And in some of these patients, MRI has revealed early avascular necrosis.

Clearly these clinical observations, "soft" though they might be, raise the possibility that anti-aggregant or anticoagulant treatment might have a place in some cases of early AVN – especially in aPL-positive patients.

17.2 Bone Fracture

An important study reported a series of Hughes Syndrome patients with "idiopathic" fracture of the metatarsal – the so-called "march fracture" traditionally seen in army recruits.

It seems probable that these fractures in the foot bones of aPL-positive individuals are also secondary to arterial ischaemia. Not surprisingly, a number of the "idiopathic" bone fractures in APS have been reported, including rib and vertebral fractures (Fig. 17.2).

17.3 Arthritis

True arthritis is rare in APS but common in lupus or Sjögren's patients with positive aPL. Thus it is likely that the complaints of widespread arthralgias in an aPL-positive person are secondary to an associated underlying connective tissue disease such as lupus, or more likely, Sjögren's Syndrome (see Chap. 23).

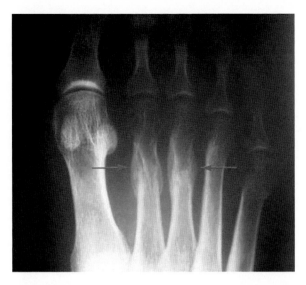

FIGURE 17.2 Non-traumatic metatarsal fractures in Hughes syndrome - multiple partially healed (callus) metatarsal fractures (*arrow*)

17.4 Reflex Dystrophy

This rare, bizarre condition, also known as "algodystrophy", is characterised by pain and swelling in a joint (such as the wrist) accompanied by overlying skin changes – shininess and tenderness.

Although the condition usually follows a relatively minor trauma, it results in severe disability, the limb being clinically "paralysed," the skin showing livedo and other possibly ischaemic changes (Fig. 17.3). The cause is unknown.

There are a small number of cases reported in APS and it is possible that an underlying ischaemic tendency such as that in APS could be a contributing factor in such cases.

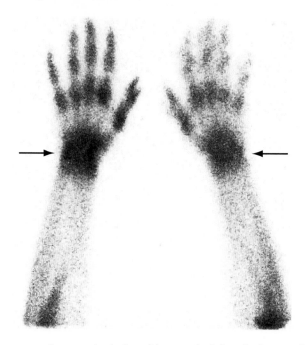

FIGURE 17.3 Increased uptake of isotope in left wrist in a patient with reflex dystrophy in Hughes syndrome. (Image reproduced with permission from Medscape.com, 2011. Available at: http://emedicine.medscape.com/article/394928-overview)

17.5 Orthopaedic Surgery

The medical and financial cost of post-operative thrombosis following knee or hip surgery is huge. Testing for thrombophilia and prophylactic anticoagulant treatment, while becoming more widespread in orthopaedic practice, is still not routine. Testing for aPL should become a standard (inexpensive) part of the routine pre-op assessment in major surgery, particularly surgery to the knee or hip.

Chapter 18
Blood

18.1 Platelets

Thrombocytopenia is an important manifestation of APS. Depending on definitions (principally the cut-off level of platelet count), thrombocytopenia has been recorded in as many as 40% of patients with APS.

The clinical picture is most commonly one of chronic, mild thrombocytopenia – for example, with platelet counts in the 90,000–120,000 range. Severe, symptomatic thrombocytopenia (e.g., under 30,000) is unusual. Having said this, "idiopathic", thrombocytopenia – ITP – can be the presenting manifestation (sometimes in childhood), of Hughes Syndrome. Likewise, studies of series of patients with ITP reveal up to 25% with positive aPL tests.

18.2 Other Platelet Manifestations

"Pseudo-thrombocytopenia" is the phenomenon where a borderline or low platelet count on an automated count is found to be higher (or even normal) on a visual count. The phenomenon is due to in vitro platelet clumping and is clinically associated with aPL, again supporting the theory that platelet membrane changes may be one mechanism in APS.

G. Hughes, S. Sangle, *Hughes Syndrome: The Antiphospholipid Syndrome*, DOI 10.1007/978-0-85729-739-6_18, © Springer-Verlag London Limited 2012

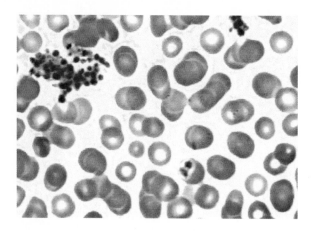

FIGURE 18.1 A peripheral blood film showing clumping of platelets in Hughes syndrome

Heparin-induced thrombocytopenia has also been reported in association with aPL. Fortunately, this has not proved a significant clinical problem with low-molecular-weight heparins, the heparin treatment of choice.

18.3 Evans Syndrome

This eponymous syndrome is the clinical association of thrombocytopenia and autoimmune haemolytic anaemia. Previously reported in up to 5% of patients with SLE, it is now recognised as being more associated with aPL, some patients going on to develop more widespread features of APS. Positive Coombs' tests are seen in some 10% of APS patients.

18.4 Thrombotic Thrombocytopenic Purpura (TTP)

TTP is a syndrome characterised by a widespread thrombic micro-angiopathy, notably affecting the CNS and kidney.

Platelets are consumed in the thrombotic process leading to thrombocytopenia and haemorrhage.

Similar pictures are seen in other thrombotic micro-angiopathies such as the haemolytic uraemic syndrome (HUS) and the HELLP syndrome (haemolysis, elevated liver enzymes, low platelets, seen in pregnancy).

The relationship between aPL and TTP is still being worked out; at present it is apparent that a (small) percentage of patients with TTP are aPL positive.

18.5 Leucopenia

Leucopaenia is common in SLE and Sjögren's – but not necessarily with aPL. Bone marrow ischaemia and infarction have been described.

Chapter 19
Catastrophic APS

19.1 Background

In the 1980s with the increasing referral pattern of APS patients to our unit, we began to see cases of acute, widespread thrombotic disease, always requiring the help of the intensive care unit and with a high fatality rate. There was no clear triggering factor, though in one of our cases, the acute collapse occurred in a patient with Hughes Syndrome, whose warfarin was stopped following a head injury.

In 1991, Greisman reported two patients with "acute catastrophic, widespread non-inflammatory visceral vascular occlusions associated with high titre antiphospholipid antibodies".

In an editorial in the same issue of the journal, my colleague Nigel Harris described two further cases. Another of my research fellows, Ron Asherson, a year later, repeated the term "catastrophic" in a series of 20 of our cases.

Thanks in large part to the efforts of Ron Asherson and Richard Cervera, an international registry of this rare "catastrophic" APS has been initiated.

19.2 Clinical Features

Approximately one half of the patients had no prior thrombotic history. In those with previous thromboses, arterial thrombosis accounted for a minority (13%).

G. Hughes, S. Sangle, *Hughes Syndrome: The Antiphospholipid Syndrome*, DOI 10.1007/978-0-85729-739-6_19,
© Springer-Verlag London Limited 2012

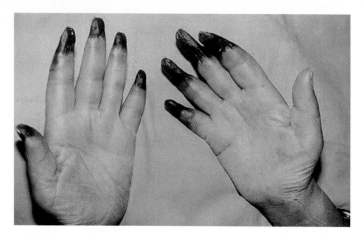

FIGURE 19.1 Catastrophic APS (Khamashta, M.A., *Hughes Syndrome: Antiphospholipid Syndrome*, 2nd ed., 2006, reproduced with permission from Springer Science+Business Media B.V.)

A prior history of miscarriage or of thrombocytopenia was rare. Precipitating factors were diverse, and included infection, recent fetal loss and surgery. However, in the majority, there was no clear trigger (Fig. 19.1).

The characteristic feature is of widespread thrombosis, including renal, cerebral, pulmonary involvement.

Clinical sequelae include adult respiratory stress syndrome, adrenal infarction (leading in some cases to Addison's disease), and seizure, livedo and widespread skin necrosis.

Thrombocytopenia occurs in approximately one half of these patients and a picture of disseminated intravascular coagulation (DIC) is seen in some. In most reported series, some 50% of cases are fatal.

19.3 Treatment

As multi-organ failure occurs, treatment always involves intensive care therapy. At the present time, the combination of heparin, steroids, plasmapheresis and IVIG seemed to provide a marginally better outcome in this extreme form of APS.

Chapter 20
Diagnosis

20.1 Introduction

The central pillar in the diagnosis of APS is the detection of antibodies against phospholipids. Two tests are routinely used, the anticardiolipin test (aCL) and the so-called lupus anticoagulant (LA).

Unfortunately, as some patients may have only one of the two tests positive, it is recommended that both tests are ordered.

20.2 Anticardiolipin Antibodies

Based on an old test for syphilis, the so-called Wasserman reaction (WR), the immunoassay for anticardiolipin (aCL), is far more sensitive and has become the most reliable and widely used test. The antibody is tested for ELISA in most labs. Unfortunately, as different ELISA kits use different recipes, there is variation from lab to lab.

Most labs measure the different classes of antibody – i.e., IgG aCL, lgM aCL and (though by no means routinely) IgA aCL.

Positive results are usually expressed as low, medium or high.

G. Hughes, S. Sangle, *Hughes Syndrome: The Antiphospholipid Syndrome*, DOI 10.1007/978-0-85729-739-6_20,
© Springer-Verlag London Limited 2012

In general, a high IgG anticardiolipin result is more of a risk factor for thrombosis than IgM, but there are many exceptions to this rule.

Positive aCL tests are reasonably specific for Hughes Syndrome, and unlike, say, anti-DNA tests in lupus, tend to remain fairly constant.

20.3 Lupus Anticoagulant (LA)

This capricious test should have been abandoned long ago. It survives partly because in some cases of APS, the only positive test is the LA. It is a rather complicated test, which indirectly measures the effects of antiphospholipid antibodies on blood clotting. To make matters worse, there are a number of different ways to measure LA, such as the direct Russel Viper Venom Time (DRVVT).

The test is also affected by treatment and cannot be interpreted if the patient is taking Warfarin. And the name is unfortunate – it is neither a "lupus" test nor an "anticoagulant" test. However, until something better comes along, the name has stuck.

20.4 Anti-Beta 2 GP1

It is now recognised that antiphospholipid antibodies don't in fact react solely with phospholipids.

[Realistically the name APS is wrong.] They react with a complex mix of phospholipid and "carrier" proteins. A number of these carrier proteins or "co-factors" are known, the most well recognised being Beta 2 GP 1 and prothrombin.

Anti-Beta 2 assays have been introduced by a number of Kit companies in an attempt to broaden the diagnostic yield.

20.5 Other Tests

Hughes Syndrome is an autoimmune disease, and other antibodies may be detected. These include ANA (common-often with accompanying Sjögren's syndrome), anti-DNA (where APS is part of lupus), thyroid antibodies and mitochondrial antibodies (type V). Coombs' tests for haemolytic anaemia may be positive.

Chapter 21
Treatment

Put at its simplest, there are three treatments for APS, aspirin, heparin and warfarin. This somewhat truncated overview, however, hides the fact that treatment can be very effective, despite the limited therapeutic armoury.

21.1 Aspirin

Because of its effects in reducing platelet stickiness, low-dose aspirin (75–100 mg daily) is extremely useful in APS. Although evidence-based data have proved rather elusive, aspirin is the drug of choice for milder cases of APS, for example, those without previous major thrombosis. It is also used as prophylaxis for aPL-positive individuals who have not had major medical problems – though studies are still ongoing. Perhaps the best data on aspirin use in aPL-positive persons have come from pregnancy studies, where low-dose aspirin in aPL-positive pregnancies has contributed to the dramatic improvement in pregnancy success rates in these women.

Clinically, the efficacy of "junior" aspirin can often be seen in the improvement in severity and frequency of migraines. However, not all patients respond. Possibly this reflects the possible different mechanisms in APS, aspirin working solely on platelets.

G. Hughes, S. Sangle, *Hughes Syndrome: The Antiphospholipid Syndrome*, DOI 10.1007/978-0-85729-739-6_21,
© Springer-Verlag London Limited 2012

A number of patients (such as asthmatics who may not be able to tolerate aspirin) respond equally well to Plavix (clopidogrel) 75 mg daily.

While there is a big literature comparing aspirin and clopidogrel in the field of cardiology, no similar comparative trials have yet been completed in APS.

Finally, dosage. Occasionally, some patients who achieve partial success on 75 mg aspirin daily appear to improve further at a dose of 150 mg daily – though these are a minority.

21.2 Heparin

Although some countries cling to old-fashioned heparin, for most centres, this has been replaced by low molecular weight (LMW) heparins (e.g., enoxaparin or dalteparin) (Fig. 21.1).

LMW heparins are well tolerated, easy to self-administer and very safe. The well-known problems of "old" heparin (e.g., heparin-induced thrombocytopenia and osteoporosis) appear to be very rare with LMW heparin.

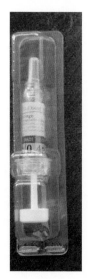

FIGURE 21.1 Low-molecular-weight heparin prefilled syringe

Heparin is widely used as first line therapy after thrombosis but has many other uses, e.g., peri-operatively or during intravenous infusions to keep the line clear.

In Hughes Syndrome, LMW heparin has found a number of other uses, including pregnancy, IVF and occasionally in diagnosis and management of some of the neurological features of APS.

In pregnancy, most specialist units use a combination of aspirin and LMW heparin in APS women with previous thrombosis and recurrent pregnancy loss, though there is still debate about best treatment.

Although heparin requires self-injection daily for several months in these pregnancies, it is surprisingly well tolerated and side effects are rare. It is no longer considered necessary to measure factor X-a levels routinely.

In neurology, we have found a short course of heparin useful as a diagnostic aid. It is not unusual for a patient with Hughes Syndrome on, say, aspirin 75 mg daily, to suffer increasingly severe hemiplegic migraines. In such a patient, with no previous history of thrombosis, warfarin treatment would seem a step too far. We have found that a standardised course of heparin – for example, Fragmin (dalteparin) 10,000 iu. daily subcutaneous for 3–4 weeks, often gives a clear idea as to whether the symptoms can be relieved by anticoagulation. While obviously a rather "soft" therapeutic trial, we have found it to be invaluable in the management of some patients.

21.3 Warfarin

For those patients with major thrombotic histories or severe neurological features such as stroke, warfarin treatment is vital.

Sadly, warfarin comes up against two widely held opinions – firstly that warfarin ("rat poison") is toxic (fortunately, apart from its effects as an anticoagulant, side effects are rare) and secondly in stroke. There is often still more of a fear of bleeding than of clotting – the danger in Hughes Syndrome is one of *clotting*.

Another problem concerns INR levels. Many patients with Hughes Syndrome require a higher INR (thinner blood) than the average anticoagulant clinic patient.

This is often especially the case with some of the neurological problems, where INR levels of 3.5–4 may be required. It is not uncommon for patients with Hughes Syndrome to "know" their INR, the headaches, dizziness and memory difficulties returning, for example, when the INR falls below, say, 3.5.

Of course warfarin control can be notoriously wayward. Patients come to clinic, for example, with a label of "unresponsive to warfarin" - in many cases a glance at the INR results shows the INR often not hitting the three level.

For this, and other reasons, it is my practice to encourage INR self-testing where possible – usually in collaboration with the anticoagulant clinic.

There are a number of self-testing kits available and most patients quickly learn the technique. A return of headaches, or dizziness, for example, quickly leading to a simple finger prick test and fine tuning, if need be, of the warfarin dose.

For many APS patients, INR self-testing has proved a liberating experience, allowing, for example, travel to other countries without fear.

21.4 Newer Anticoagulants

For some years, there has been a hope of newer anticoagulants, which hopefully don't require injection, or INR testing. Some have fallen by the wayside in early trials, but one or two (e.g., debigatran – Pradaxa) are very promising and will hopefully prove of value in some cases of APS.

21.5 Steroids

Steroids are not indicated for thrombosis problems. However, they are still one of the first choices for the treatment of thrombocytopenia. They are also a part of the treatment of lupus, including those lupus patients with aPL-associated problems.

21.6 Immunosuppressives

Because Hughes Syndrome is an "auto-immune" condition, it seemed logical to attempt to address the problem of an over-active immune system.

Unfortunately, our early attempts at immunosuppressives – usually with azathioprine and cyclophosphamide – were disappointing and seemed to have little impact on the disease.

More recently, newer "selective" immunosuppressants, such as the anti-B cell agents rituximab and belimumab, have proved very promising in a number of autoimmune conditions such as lupus, and anecdotally, and in small numbers, positive reports in Hughes Syndrome are appearing. Early days!

Chapter 22
Hughes Syndrome: The Causes – Genetics Versus Environment

22.1 Introduction

Hughes Syndrome is a result of altered immunity. In this instance a family of antibodies – aPL – are closely linked to the disease process. It is still not proven whether this is a cause-and-effect link (e.g., altered phospholipid-membrane structure in platelets and endothelial cells), but the suspicion is there.

As in other "autoimmune" diseases, there is evidence that both genetic and environmental influences are implicated.

22.2 Autoimmunity

The evidence for an autoimmune label comes from a number of sources – the association with other autoimmune conditions such as lupus, Sjögren's and Hashimoto's thyroiditis, for example, and the frequent finding of other clues – the presence of other antibodies such as ANA, the frequent hyperglobulinemia and the often high titres of antiphospholipid antibody.

With the advent of newer immunosuppressives such as the anti-B cell drugs rituximab and belimumab, some early successes have also, indirectly, pointed to the immune nature of the illness.

G. Hughes, S. Sangle, *Hughes Syndrome: The Antiphospholipid Syndrome*, DOI 10.1007/978-0-85729-739-6_22,
© Springer-Verlag London Limited 2012

22.3 Clotting

Whatever the links between B cells, antibody and disease, the end result is thrombosis – both venous and, strikingly, arterial. Studies of the effects of aPL, both in man and mice, have shown aPL-related changes in platelets, in endothelial cell function and in the clotting cascade itself.

It is possible that further analysis of the relative importance of each mechanism might provide more targeted treatment.

22.4 Genetics

Clinical experience has shown that families exist with multiple members with APS. And not only with APS, but with other related conditions – for example, families with clotting, thyroid disease, migraine and multiple sclerosis.

To date, HLA and related studies have had mixed results. Some studies showed an increased frequency of HLA DR4, others DRB1 0402 and DQB1 0302.

However, a number of factors, ranging from patient inclusion to antigen heterogeneity, make risk factor determination difficult.

22.5 Environmental Factors

Arterial (and possibly venous) disease is clearly affected by environmental factors such as lifestyle, diet, stress and so on. Likewise, APS is influenced by outside factors – especially factors which themselves can possibly predispose to thrombosis.

22.5.1 Diet

An interesting study compared patients in India and in Kuwait. The same physician (Dr. Malaviya) worked in both countries and studied Hughes Syndrome. It turned out that the prevalence of aPL – the antibody – was similar in both countries. However, the incidence of thrombosis was far greater in Kuwait. Dr. Malaviya suggested that lifestyle differences (vegetarian in India, for example) could affect the phenotypic expression of the disease.

22.5.2 The Pill

As might be expected, the oral contraceptive (and smoking) has been shown to increase the risk of thrombosis in aPL-positive women. In one large study of aPL-positive women smokers, under-50, the odds ratio on developing a stroke, on starting the oral contraceptive pill, was increased 200 times! In a number of patients, the initial clinical manifestations of Hughes Syndrome (e.g., migraine or even stroke) appear when the oral contraceptive pill is started. Thus it seems reasonable to avoid oestrogen supplementation in aPL-positive women – indeed, aPL testing could be recommended in any young women with possible aPL risk factors, such as positive family history.

22.5.3 Infection

In some patients (especially in children where diarrhoeal illness can lead to dehydration), infections seem to trigger a thrombotic event – indeed, infectious triggers are often cited in the catastrophic APS. The list of infections implicated is long and varied.

However, the link remains unproven – in fact, most APS patients seem to deal normally with common infections such as colds, coughs, flu and chest and urinary infections.

22.5.4 Altitude

A number of patients with Hughes Syndrome are badly affected by altitude, with increasing headaches at higher mountain heights.

One aPL-positive young man became comatose whilst climbing in the Andes (Case 41 - Hughes (2009) Understanding Hughes Syndrome - case studies for patients (Publisher: Springer).

Of course, there is a substantial literature on altitude sickness, which includes seizures, strokes and coma. There are no data as yet on the relative risk (if any) in aPL-positive individuals.

22.6 Economy Class Syndrome

This term arose following publicity around a number of cases of thrombosis (notably DVT) in passengers on long haul flights – especially those in cramped conditions. Obviously the risk is not confined to aeroplanes, but the name stuck.

Is there an increased risk for aPL-positive individuals? Anecdotally, a number of APS patients have suffered DVT after long haul flights – it seems logical to suppose that aPL does confer an increased risk in under-treated individuals.

An interesting observation has come to light. A number of patients with Hughes Syndrome complain of felling unwell for a few days after a long flight, common symptoms being headache, balance problems and fatigue. And a number of these individuals have found that the problem doesn't happen if an injection of low-molecular-weight heparin is taken before the flight.

Placebo perhaps, but I believe the observation is sufficiently frequent to warrant further investigation. Cabin pressures, whilst reasonable, can fall, especially when engine power is reduced at the start of descent.

Chapter 23
Links to Other Diseases

Firstly, it is important to point out that primary APS rarely metamorphoses into other diseases. Many patients are concerned that in future they may develop lupus (not helped by the unfortunately named "lupus–anticoagulant" test). Unless the evidence of lupus (or Sjögren's) is already present at diagnosis, progression or "widening" of the disease is very unusual.

23.1 Lupus

Figure 23.1 shows in "Venn diagram" form the relationship between APS and lupus. Many of us believe that the "APS circle" will continue to enlarge, to become considerably greater than lupus, as more cases become diagnosed.

Depending on the sensitivity of the tests used, up to 1 in 5 lupus patients demonstrate positive tests for aPL. Many of these patients also develop features of APS – often referred to as "secondary APS".

A number of studies have shown that there is little difference between primary APS and the APS associated with conditions such as lupus.

For patients with lupus however, the discovery of the antiphospholipid syndrome has totally revolutionised the management of the disease. Many features such as seizures,

G. Hughes, S. Sangle, *Hughes Syndrome: The Antiphospholipid Syndrome*, DOI 10.1007/978-0-85729-739-6_23,
© Springer-Verlag London Limited 2012

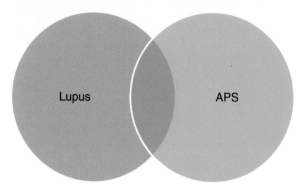

FIGURE 23.1 Hughes syndrome is often associated with other autoimmune diseases such as Lupus/Sjögren's Syndrome

visual loss, stroke and transverse myelitis can just as possibly be due to thrombosis as to inflammation – such cases possibly requiring anticoagulation rather than more and more steroids.

23.2 Sjögren's Syndrome

Sjögren's syndrome, originally a triad of dry eyes, dry mouth and arthritis, is now recognised as an important, common condition.

A disease characterised by an overactive immune system, it occupies a central place in the connective tissue disease spectrum, linking the organ-specific disorder (thyroid, celiac, pernicious anaemia) with the non-organ-specific antibody diseases (lupus, rheumatoid arthritis).

A simple clinical test for Sjögren's syndrome is the Schirmer tear test – the degree of moistening of a standardised "blotter" strip. Although the test is "crude", it is extremely useful. While normal individuals wet the blotting paper strip in seconds, Sjögren's patients remain "dry", even at 5 min (see chap. 13 fig. 13.3).

Why is Sjögren's important? It is clinically important for at least two reasons.

Firstly, because it accounts for many of the clinical symptoms seen in the broad family of autoimmune conditions – fatigue, aches and pains, allergies, photosensitivity, raised gamma-globulins, positive ANA – and so on.

And secondly, it links disorders such as Hughes Syndrome to other autoimmune disorders such as hypothyroidism and celiac disease – often explaining some of the puzzling features seen in individual patients attending clinic.

23.3 Other Diseases

Crohn's disease – inflammatory bowel disease, perhaps strangely (it has few, if any, "autoimmune" features), sometimes has both positive aPL as well as clinical features of APS – headaches, migraine, thrombosis. Somewhat surprisingly, aPL and APS are unusual in rheumatoid, scleroderma and myositis.

23.4 Seronegative APS

A number of patients are seen with some of the "classical" features of APS – arterial thrombosis, valve disease, thrombocytopenia, recurrent miscarriage, in whom conventional aPL testing is negative. Even more supportive of the diagnosis, for example, can be the positive family history of thrombosis and autoimmune disease.

There are three possible explanations for "seronegative" APS. Firstly, the diagnosis may be wrong. Secondly, that previous positive aPL are now negative (it *can* happen). Thirdly, that new more sensitive tests are needed.

The "seronegative" concept is important. Years ago, it opened our eyes to clinically important variants both in rheumatoid arthritis and in lupus.

Chapter 24
Conclusions: The World Map

24.1 Thirty Years Old

Although the description of the syndrome, its critical propensity to artery thrombosis (e.g. stroke) and the development of simple assays for its detection are "modern" in comparative medical terms, for some of us, progress seems slow. For example, in a recent, "YouGov", survey, commissioned by the charity, Hughes Syndrome Foundation (www.hughes-syndromefoundation.co.uk), only 15% of the responding public had heard of Hughes Syndrome or APS.

Yet there are grounds for optimism. In the world of obstetrics, aPL testing after serial miscarriage and late pregnancy loss is becoming standard practice.

24.2 One in Five

A rough rule of thumb can be drawn from publications so far, relating to Hughes Syndrome (APS) (Fig. 24.1).

Hughes Syndrome accounts for 1 in 5 of all cases of recurrent miscarriage.

It accounts for 1 in 5 cases of DVT.

It accounts for 1 in 5 cases of stroke in the under 45 year olds – a striking figure!

And in lupus? Some 1 in 5 have positive aPL tests, with the consequent thrombotic complications.

G. Hughes, S. Sangle, *Hughes Syndrome: The Antiphospholipid Syndrome*, DOI 10.1007/978-0-85729-739-6_24,

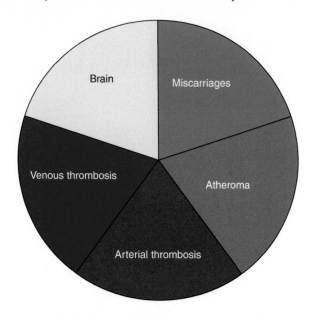

FIGURE 24.1 Major features of HS

24.3 Also One in Five?

Recent reports have suggested that young (under 45) patients – particularly females – with myocardial infarction have underlying Hughes Syndrome – 40% in one series having positive tests for aPL.

In the world of neurology, epilepsy has been shown to be an important feature – one study showing that 1 in 5 cases of ideopathic teenage epilepsy were aPL positive.

24.4 Migraine

Perhaps the biggest "missing link" concerns migraine. Such a common and prominent symptom in so many Hughes Syndrome patients, migraine, in all its forms, has received surprisingly few major studies linking it with APS.

Yet the literature contains a significant number of reports linking migraine with stroke and with heart attack. This physician believes that APS could be a strong "missing link" between migraine and vascular disease.

24.5 What Else?

Bright students of medicine will have picked up on a number of leads, published in the literature, picked up in this short book, which "need further study". Some are highlighted here.

24.6 The Pill

The danger of thrombosis on the oral contraceptive pill is well known. The significantly increased risk of an aPL-positive woman developing thrombosis on the pill is not.

The report that an aPL-positive woman smoker starting the oral contraceptive has a 200-fold increase of suffering a stroke and a 20-fold increased risk of heart attack is arresting and vitally important.

24.7 Orthopaedic Surgery

DVT following knee or hip surgery costs every country millions of pounds. Many orthopaedic units now carry out pre-operative blood tests for clotting tendencies such as Factor V Leiden deficiency and aPL – but not all.

Furthermore, the discovery that some cases of unexpected fracture and of hip necrosis could be due to ischaemia secondary to Hughes Syndrome opens up important lines of research.

24.8 Memory Loss

In the longer term, it may well be that memory loss will become the leading clinical feature of Hughes Syndrome. Certainly in clinical practice, it is a common and extremely

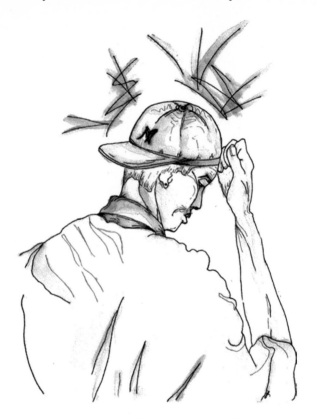

FIGURE 24.2 Memory loss in HS (Reproduced with kind permission from Understanding Hughes Syndrome, ISBN-978-1-84800-375-09 Springer)

worrying symptom in Hughes Syndrome patients (Fig. 24.2).

In busy clinical practice however, there is not the time, nor the personnel for in-depth memory and other psychiatric testing.

Yet this is one of the potentially most important findings of the syndrome – a serious, yet potentially reversible brain problem – an aspect of Hughes Syndrome which, with future careful psychometric studies, must come to be recognised for the important clinical symptom that it surely is.

24.9 Unexpected Fracture

Again, the reports of metatarsal fractures in some patients with Hughes Syndrome may turn out to be the tip of the iceberg. Already there are reports of other fractures – possibly on the basis of bone ischaemia.

Those working in osteoporosis have long recognised that some patients seem to fracture without evidence of demineralisation – perhaps a percentage of these will prove to have "sticky blood".

24.10 Infertility

We hope that the next few years might provide more insights into a possible link between antiphospholipid antibodies (aPL) and infertility. There are a number of excellent research groups looking at aPL and their influence on placentation, embryogenesis and vascular supply in each pregnancy.

24.11 And in Lupus?

In my own subject, lupus, the discovery of the antiphospholipid syndrome has genuinely revolutionised management. Many lupus features previously thought to be inflammatory – and "steroid-requiring" – are now thought more likely to be due to aPL-related thrombosis.

In the brain, for example, many features previously thought to be inflammatory, "vasculitis" – including stroke, seizure, myelopathy, memory loss, visual disturbance – are almost certainly more likely to be aPL related.

In the kidney, one of the major indications for renal biopsy is to assess the extent of glomerular thrombosis.

In pregnancy, we now know that lupus itself is almost certainly *not* a cause of miscarriage – it is the subset with aPL who are at risk.

And in treatment, the description of the syndrome has tipped the focus just a little bit away from steroids and immunosuppressives towards a more logical consideration in some cases of aspirin, heparin or warfarin.

24.12 Education

The recent, "YouGov", survey showed, as might be expected, that few members of the general public were aware of APS/Hughes Syndrome. Hopefully, this will change.

I remember a similar survey 40 years ago conducted by a TV company asking about awareness of lupus. Few of those interviewed in Trafalgar Square had ever heard of lupus. How *that* has changed!

Index

G. Hughes, S. Sangle, *Hughes Syndrome: The Antiphospholipid*   99
Syndrome, DOI 10.1007/978-0-85729-739-6
© Springer-Verlag London Limited 2012